Wellness Wonders

The Transformative Power of THC, CBD, CBG, and CBH

A short introduction by The HealthSpan Institute

Wellness Wonders:
The Transformative Power of THC, CBD, CBG, and CBH

ISBN: 9798876192233

Copyright © 2024 Wellness Press

Printed in the United States of America

Contents

Chapter 1: Introduction to Cannabinoids

Chapter 2:
THC – The Trailblazer

Chapter 3:
CBD – The Wellness Warrior

Chapter 4:
CBG – The Rising Star

Chapter 5:
CBH – The New Frontier

Chapter 6:
Synergistic Effects and the Entourage Effect

Chapter 7:
Future Directions and Challenges

Chapter 1: Introduction to Cannabinoids

Understanding Cannabinoids: THC, CBD, CBG, and CBH

Cannabinoids, the active chemical compounds found in the cannabis plant, have recently gained significant attention in the medical and wellness communities. Among these, Tetrahydrocannabinol (THC), Cannabidiol (CBD), Cannabigerol (CBG), and Cannabihexol (CBH) stand out for their unique properties and potential health benefits. This section delves into the nature, characteristics, and the therapeutic potential of these fascinating compounds.

The Nature of Cannabinoids

Cannabinoids are part of a complex chemical group found predominantly in the cannabis plant. These compounds interact with the body's endocannabinoid system (ECS), a vast network of receptors and neurotransmitters that play a crucial role in maintaining homeostasis. The ECS influences various physiological processes including mood, pain sensation, appetite, and memory. THC, CBD, CBG, and CBH, each interact with the ECS in different ways, leading to a variety of effects and potential benefits.

Tetrahydrocannabinol (THC)

THC is the most well-known cannabinoid due to its psychoactive effects. It binds primarily to the CB1 receptors in the brain, producing the 'high' associated with cannabis. However, THC's impact goes beyond recreational use. It has shown promise in treating chronic pain, nausea, and muscle spasms. Additionally, THC has been used to increase appetite in patients undergoing chemotherapy and those with AIDS.

Cannabidiol (CBD)

CBD has surged in popularity, primarily due to its non-psychoactive nature. Unlike THC, CBD does not produce a high and has a more indirect interaction with the ECS. It is known for its anti-inflammatory, anti-anxiety, and anti-seizure properties. CBD has been particularly noted for its effectiveness in treating epilepsy, as evidenced by the FDA-approved drug Epidiolex. It also shows potential in treating anxiety disorders, chronic pain, and even has implications in cardiovascular health.

Cannabigerol (CBG)

CBG, though less researched, is emerging as a cannabinoid with significant therapeutic potential. Often referred to as the 'mother of all cannabinoids,' it is the precursor from which other cannabinoids are synthesized. Early studies suggest that CBG may have anti-inflammatory, anti-bacterial, and neuroprotective properties. It holds potential in treating conditions like inflammatory bowel disease, glaucoma, and even certain neurological disorders.

Cannabihexol (CBH)

CBH is one of the newer cannabinoids to be identified and remains the least understood. Its rarity in the cannabis plant makes research challenging. Preliminary studies indicate that it may possess unique properties that differentiate it from its more famous counterparts. The potential medical applications of CBH are still being explored, with early indications suggesting it might offer benefits not found in other cannabinoids.

Synergistic Effects and Future Research

An exciting area of cannabinoid research is the study of how these compounds interact synergistically, often referred to as the 'entourage effect.' This theory suggests that the therapeutic impact of the whole cannabis plant is greater than the sum of its parts. Understanding how THC, CBD, CBG, and CBH work together could unlock new pathways in treatment methodologies.

In conclusion, the world of cannabinoids is rich and complex. THC, CBD, CBG, and CBH each offer unique properties and potential health benefits. As research progresses, these compounds may well redefine approaches to wellness and medicine. The ongoing exploration into the therapeutic applications of cannabinoids holds promise for new treatments and a deeper understanding of human physiology.

The History of Cannabinoid Research

The history of cannabinoid research is a fascinating journey that spans several decades, revealing how these compounds shifted from obscurity to become a focal point in modern medicinal science. This journey is not just about the discovery of individual cannabinoids like THC, CBD, CBG, and CBH, but also about understanding their effects, potential therapeutic applications, and the evolving legal and social attitudes towards them.

Early Discoveries and Isolation of Cannabinoids

Cannabinoid research effectively began in the early 20th century, but the use of cannabis for medicinal purposes dates back thousands of years. Ancient texts from China, Egypt, and India mention the use of cannabis for a variety of ailments. However, it wasn't until the 1940s that the first cannabinoid, Cannabinol (CBN), was isolated. This was followed by the isolation of CBD in 1942 and THC in 1964 by Raphael Mechoulam and Yechiel Gaoni at the Weizmann Institute of Science in Israel, marking a significant breakthrough in cannabinoid research.

Understanding the Mechanisms: The Endocannabinoid System

The discovery of THC led to an increased interest in understanding how cannabinoids interact with the human body. This quest led to one of the most significant breakthroughs in the late 1980s and early 1990s: the discovery of the endocannabinoid system (ECS).

The ECS is a complex cell-signaling system that plays a key role in regulating a range of functions and processes, including mood, appetite, memory, and pain. Understanding the ECS was crucial in comprehending how cannabinoids exert their effects.

Therapeutic Applications and Clinical Trials

Following these discoveries, the focus shifted towards exploring the therapeutic potential of cannabinoids. In the late 20th century, research began to uncover the benefits of THC and CBD in treating conditions like nausea and vomiting in chemotherapy patients, chronic pain, and severe forms of epilepsy. This period saw the development of synthetic cannabinoid-based medications such as Marinol and Epidiolex, which received FDA approval for specific medical uses.

The Emergence of CBG and CBH

While THC and CBD dominated most of the early research, the last two decades have seen increased interest in lesser-known cannabinoids like CBG and CBH. CBG, often referred to as the 'mother cannabinoid,' has shown promise in preliminary studies for its potential neuroprotective and anti-inflammatory properties. CBH, a relatively new discovery, is still in the early stages of research but is believed to have unique characteristics that could lead to new therapeutic applications.

Challenges and Controversies

Cannabinoid research has not been without its challenges. Legal restrictions on cannabis and its derivatives have historically hampered scientific study. The classification of cannabis as a Schedule I drug in many countries, including the United States, made it difficult for researchers to access high-quality cannabis for study purposes. Additionally, the social stigma associated with cannabis use has often overshadowed the scientific discourse.

Recent Developments and Future Directions

In recent years, there has been a significant shift in both legal frameworks and public opinion regarding cannabis and cannabinoids. This change has been partly driven by the growing body of research demonstrating the potential medical benefits of cannabinoids. As a result, many countries have begun to legalize cannabis for medical and even recreational use, paving the way for more comprehensive and groundbreaking research.

The future of cannabinoid research looks promising. The ongoing exploration of the ECS and the potential synergistic effects of different cannabinoids (the 'entourage effect') could lead to the development of more effective and targeted therapies. Research into the therapeutic applications of CBG and CBH is particularly exciting, as these compounds may offer new benefits and mechanisms of action that are currently unknown.

Moreover, advancements in technology and methodology are allowing for more precise and detailed study of cannabinoids. Sophisticated extraction techniques, genetic engineering, and better analytical tools are enabling researchers to isolate cannabinoids more efficiently and study them in greater depth.

One of the most promising areas of research is the use of cannabinoids in neurology. Studies are exploring the potential of cannabinoids in treating conditions like Alzheimer's disease, Parkinson's disease, and multiple sclerosis. The neuroprotective properties of cannabinoids, particularly CBG, are of significant interest, as they may offer a pathway to treatments for neurodegenerative disorders.

The potential of cannabinoids in oncology is also an area of intense study. Preliminary research suggests that certain cannabinoids may have anti-cancer properties. While much of this research is still in its infancy, it opens up exciting possibilities for the use of cannabinoids in cancer treatment.

The challenges in cannabinoid research remain, primarily in standardizing and regulating cannabinoid-based treatments. The variability in cannabis plant strains, extraction methods, and individual responses makes it difficult to create consistent and reliable medications. Furthermore, the need for more comprehensive clinical trials to establish efficacy, dosage, and safety is paramount.

In conclusion, the history of cannabinoid research is a testament to the evolving understanding of medicinal plants and their potential in modern medicine. From the early isolation of cannabinoids to the current exploration of their therapeutic applications, this field has continually challenged and expanded our knowledge of pharmacology and human biology. As research continues to advance, it promises not only new treatments but also a deeper understanding of the complex interplay between natural compounds and human health.

Legal and Cultural Perspectives on Cannabinoids

The journey of cannabinoids, particularly THC, CBD, CBG, and CBH, through the landscape of legal and cultural perspectives has been complex and dynamic. This section explores the evolution of societal attitudes, legal frameworks, and cultural implications surrounding these substances, highlighting the significant shifts that have influenced both policy and public perception.

Historical Context and Early Attitudes

Cannabinoids have a long history that intertwines with human cultures. For centuries, cannabis, the plant from which these compounds are derived, was used for medicinal, spiritual, and recreational purposes in various cultures. However, the 20th century marked a turning point, with a growing stigma surrounding cannabis use, largely due to misconceptions and politicized narratives. This led to stringent regulations worldwide, with many countries criminalizing cannabis and its derivatives.

The War on Drugs and Its Impact

The "War on Drugs," initiated in the United States in the 1970s, significantly impacted the legal status of cannabis. This campaign, aimed at reducing drug use, resulted in strict laws and severe penalties for cannabis possession and use. The classification of cannabis as a Schedule I drug, alongside substances like heroin and LSD, reflected a period of heightened skepticism and aversion towards cannabinoids, impeding both use and research.

Shift in Perceptions and Legalization Movements

In the late 20th and early 21st centuries, a gradual shift occurred in the perception of cannabinoids. This change was driven by emerging scientific research demonstrating the therapeutic potential of compounds like CBD and THC, challenging the prevailing narratives. Advocacy groups and patients began to push for the legalization of cannabis, especially for medicinal purposes. This movement gained momentum, leading to significant legal changes in various countries and states.

Medical Marijuana and CBD Legalization

The medical marijuana movement played a crucial role in changing legal perspectives. Pioneering states like California, which legalized medical marijuana in 1996, set a precedent that many others followed. The recognition of the medical benefits of cannabinoids, particularly CBD, led to a broader acceptance and legalization. The FDA approval of Epidiolex, a CBD-based medication for epilepsy, was a landmark moment, signifying the therapeutic legitimacy of cannabinoids.

The Complex Landscape of Recreational Cannabis

The legalization of recreational cannabis further complicated the legal and cultural landscape. Countries like Canada and Uruguay, along with several U.S. states, legalized recreational cannabis, reflecting a significant shift in societal attitudes. However, this shift also brought challenges in regulation, public health concerns, and ongoing debates about the implications of recreational use.

Cultural Integration and Ongoing Stigmatization

Cannabinoids, especially CBD, have seen a surge in cultural integration, appearing in a wide range of products from wellness supplements to cosmetics. This mainstream acceptance contrasts with the ongoing stigmatization in certain regions and demographics, highlighting the diverse and often conflicting cultural perspectives on cannabinoids.

International Perspectives and Policies

Globally, the approach to cannabinoids varies significantly. While some countries have embraced medicinal and even recreational cannabis, others maintain strict prohibitionist policies. This disparity reflects diverse cultural, legal, and political landscapes, influencing both the availability of cannabinoid-based treatments and the scope of research.

Future Directions and Challenges

Looking forward, the legal and cultural landscapes surrounding cannabinoids are likely to continue evolving. Key challenges include balancing regulation with accessibility, addressing public health concerns, and navigating the complex interplay between federal and state laws, particularly in the United States. Additionally, the need for further research and education to dispel myths and inform evidence-based policies remains critical.

In conclusion, the legal and cultural perspectives on cannabinoids have undergone significant transformation, driven by scientific discoveries, societal changes, and advocacy. This evolution reflects a broader shift towards a more nuanced understanding of these compounds and their place in society. As legal frameworks continue to adapt, and cultural perceptions evolve, the future of cannabinoids holds both promise and complexity.

Chapter 2:
THC – The Trailblazer

The Psychoactive World of THC

Tetrahydrocannabinol, commonly known as THC, is the most well-known and studied cannabinoid due to its psychoactive properties. This section explores the psychoactive world of THC, its effects on the human body and mind, its role in culture and medicine, and the ongoing research that continues to unravel its complexities.

Understanding THC's Psychoactive Effects

THC is renowned for its ability to alter consciousness, mood, and perception. When consumed, THC binds to cannabinoid receptors in the brain, particularly the CB1 receptors, which are abundant in regions responsible for memory, cognition, pleasure, and coordination. This interaction triggers the release of dopamine, leading to the euphoria or 'high' often associated with cannabis use. THC's psychoactive effects vary greatly among individuals and are influenced by factors such as dosage, strain, and the user's physiology and tolerance.

THC in Medical Use

Despite its psychoactive nature, THC has significant medical benefits. It has been effectively used to alleviate chronic pain, reduce nausea and vomiting in chemotherapy patients, and stimulate appetite in individuals suffering from AIDS or cancer. The psychoactive effects of THC, which can include relaxation and altered sensory perception, are also considered therapeutic for some patients, particularly those dealing with anxiety or PTSD.

The Cultural Impact of THC

THC has had a profound impact on culture, particularly in the realms of music, art, and literature, where it has been both vilified and celebrated. In the 1960s and 70s, THC and cannabis became symbols of counterculture, associated with anti-establishment movements and artistic expression. This cultural significance has evolved, with THC now being more widely accepted and integrated into mainstream culture, although it still carries a degree of controversy due to its psychoactive effects and legal status.

Recreational Use and Public Perception

The recreational use of THC has been a subject of public interest and debate. While many enjoy its psychoactive effects for relaxation and entertainment, concerns about dependency, impaired judgment, and potential long-term cognitive effects remain. Public perception of THC is deeply intertwined with its legal status, with legalization in some regions leading to a more positive view and increased acceptance.

Research and Understanding of THC's Effects

Scientific research into THC has been pivotal in understanding its effects on the human brain and body. Studies have explored how THC impacts cognitive functions, memory, motor skills, and perception. Research has also delved into the potential risks associated with THC use, such as the development of cannabis use disorder, its impact on adolescent brain development, and the association with certain mental health conditions.

THC's Role in the Endocannabinoid System

THC's interaction with the endocannabinoid system (ECS) is a key area of research. The ECS plays a crucial role in regulating various physiological processes, and THC's ability to mimic endocannabinoids and bind to ECS receptors is central to both its therapeutic and psychoactive effects. Understanding this interaction is crucial for developing targeted treatments that harness THC's benefits while minimizing adverse effects.

Legal Challenges and Future Research

The legal status of THC remains a significant hurdle for research. In many regions, strict regulations on cannabis and THC impede scientific study, limiting the understanding of its full potential and risks. As legalization movements gain traction, there is hope for more comprehensive research that can guide policy and inform safe, effective medical use.

In conclusion, THC's psychoactive world is complex and multi-faceted, encompassing medical, cultural, and recreational dimensions. Its ability to alter perception and mood has made it a subject of fascination, controversy, and significant scientific interest. As research continues to advance, our understanding of THC will

become more nuanced, potentially leading to new therapeutic applications and a deeper appreciation of its role in both culture and medicine.

The psychoactive properties of THC, while often the focus of public discourse, represent just one aspect of this cannabinoid's impact. Its medicinal benefits are increasingly recognized, offering relief for a variety of conditions. Moreover, the cultural and social dimensions of THC reflect broader societal attitudes towards cannabis and drug policy.

As we move forward, the challenge lies in balancing the enjoyment of THC's psychoactive properties with responsible use and understanding its potential risks. Education plays a crucial role in this, helping individuals make informed choices about their use of THC and cannabis in general.

Furthermore, the legal landscape surrounding THC is likely to continue evolving. This will have a significant impact on both the availability of THC for medicinal and recreational purposes and the scope of research into its effects and potential uses. Navigating these legal changes, while ensuring public safety and health, remains a key challenge for policymakers and healthcare professionals.

The future of THC research holds great promise. Advances in our understanding of the ECS and the development of new cannabis strains with varying THC levels open up exciting possibilities for both medical and recreational use. Research into THC's long-term effects, particularly on the developing brain, is crucial for guiding its safe use.

In summary, the world of THC is a rich tapestry of psychoactive effects, medical potential, cultural significance, and evolving legal status. It represents a unique intersection of science, medicine, society, and law. As we continue to explore and understand THC, it will undoubtedly play a significant role in shaping future discussions and policies around cannabis and cannabinoid-based therapies.

Medical Benefits of THC

Tetrahydrocannabinol (THC), best known for its psychoactive properties, also possesses a range of therapeutic benefits that have become a focal point in modern medicinal cannabis research. This section explores the various medical benefits of THC, examining its efficacy and potential applications in treating numerous health conditions.

Pain Management

One of the most well-documented medical uses of THC is in pain management. THC has been found effective in alleviating chronic pain, neuropathic pain, and pain associated with conditions like multiple sclerosis and arthritis. It works by binding to cannabinoid receptors in the brain and nervous system, altering pain perception and providing relief. For many patients, THC-based treatments offer an alternative to traditional painkillers, particularly opioids, which have a high risk of dependency and adverse side effects.

Cancer-Related Symptoms

THC plays a significant role in managing cancer-related symptoms, particularly chemotherapy-induced nausea and vomiting. Studies have shown that THC can be more effective than some traditional antiemetic medications. Additionally, THC is known to stimulate appetite, which can be beneficial for cancer patients struggling with weight loss and malnutrition. There is also growing interest in the potential of THC to exert anti-tumor effects, although this area of research is still in its early stages.

Neurological Disorders and Spasticity

Patients with neurological disorders such as multiple sclerosis often experience muscle spasticity – painful and uncontrollable muscle contractions. THC has been shown to reduce spasticity and associated pain effectively. Its neuroprotective properties are also being explored in conditions like Parkinson's disease and Alzheimer's disease, with early research suggesting that THC may help in managing symptoms and possibly slowing disease progression.

Mental Health Conditions

The use of THC in treating certain mental health conditions is a growing area of interest. While there is controversy surrounding the relationship between THC and mental health, some studies suggest benefits in treating conditions like PTSD and anxiety. THC's ability to reduce anxiety and promote relaxation is well-documented, although it is crucial to approach this area cautiously due to the complex effects of THC on mental health.

Sleep Disorders

THC has been found to be effective in treating certain sleep disorders, such as insomnia. It can promote relaxation and reduce the time it takes to fall asleep. Additionally, THC's impact on REM sleep can be beneficial for individuals with PTSD, as it can reduce nightmares and night terrors. However, the long-term impact of THC on sleep patterns requires further study.

Autoimmune Diseases and Inflammation

THC's anti-inflammatory properties are being explored in the treatment of autoimmune diseases like Crohn's disease and rheumatoid arthritis. By interacting with the ECS, THC can help modulate the immune system and reduce inflammation, providing relief from symptoms and potentially influencing disease progression.

Challenges and Considerations in THC-Based Treatments

While the medical benefits of THC are promising, there are challenges and considerations in its use as a treatment. The psychoactive effects of THC can be a barrier for some patients, and there is a need for careful dosing to balance therapeutic benefits with potential side effects. The variability in individual responses to THC also poses a challenge, necessitating personalized treatment approaches.

Legal and Regulatory Aspects

The legal status of THC significantly impacts its availability for medical use. In regions where cannabis is legal for medicinal purposes, patients have better access to THC-based treatments. However, in areas where cannabis is still illegal, patients may lack access to these potentially beneficial therapies. The evolving legal landscape is therefore a critical factor in the future of THC as a medicine.

In conclusion, THC offers a wide range of medical benefits, making it a valuable component of the medicinal cannabis landscape. Its efficacy in pain management, alleviation of cancer-related symptoms, and potential in treating neurological and mental health disorders underscores its therapeutic significance. However, the use of THC in medicine is not without its challenges. The psychoactive effects, the need for precise dosing, and individual variability in response all necessitate a cautious and informed approach to its use.

Moreover, the legal and regulatory environment continues to play a crucial role in determining the availability and research of THC-based treatments. As laws and perceptions around cannabis continue to evolve, it is likely that the role of THC in medicine will become more prominent and better understood.

The future of THC in the medical world is promising but requires ongoing research to fully understand its potential and limitations.

Studies focusing on long-term effects, optimal dosing, and the development of formulations that minimize psychoactive effects while maximizing therapeutic benefits are essential. Additionally, exploring THC's potential in combination with other cannabinoids and treatments could open new avenues for comprehensive and effective healthcare solutions.

In summary, THC's medical benefits are a testament to the therapeutic potential of cannabinoids. As our understanding of THC continues to grow, so does the possibility of harnessing its properties for a wide range of medical applications, offering hope and relief to many patients worldwide.

Risks and Misconceptions of THC

While Tetrahydrocannabinol (THC) is celebrated for its medicinal benefits and psychoactive properties, it is also subject to various risks and misconceptions. Understanding these risks and dispelling the myths is crucial for informed use and effective regulation. This section delves into the potential risks associated with THC use and addresses common misconceptions, providing a balanced perspective.

Potential Health Risks of THC

THC use is not without potential health risks, particularly when used irresponsibly or by vulnerable populations. Among the most significant concerns are:

1. **Mental Health Risks:** High doses of THC have been linked to an increased risk of psychiatric symptoms, particularly in individuals with a pre-existing susceptibility to mental health disorders. Conditions such as schizophrenia and psychosis have been associated with high-THC cannabis use, especially in adolescents.

2. **Cognitive Impairments:** Chronic use of THC, particularly at high doses, can lead to cognitive impairments. This includes issues with memory, concentration, and decision-making.

These effects are more pronounced in individuals who start using cannabis at a young age.

3. **Dependency and Addiction:** Although less addictive than many other substances, THC can lead to dependency, particularly in those with a history of substance abuse. Withdrawal symptoms, such as irritability, mood changes, and sleep disturbances, can occur in chronic users who stop consumption.

4. **Respiratory Issues:** Smoking cannabis, like smoking tobacco, can have adverse effects on lung health. It can lead to respiratory issues, including chronic bronchitis and, in some cases, impair lung function.

Misconceptions about THC

Alongside the risks, numerous misconceptions about THC have contributed to its stigmatization and skewed public perception. Some of these misconceptions include:

1. **"THC Is Completely Harmless":** While THC has therapeutic benefits, claiming it is entirely without risk is misleading. As with any psychoactive substance, it has potential side effects and can interact differently with individual physiology.

2. **"All Cannabis Use Leads to High THC Exposure":** Not all cannabis strains or products have high THC levels. There are many strains and products, especially those designed for medical use, that have low THC and high CBD content, reducing psychoactive effects.

3. **"THC Is the Only Beneficial Cannabinoid":** While THC is one of the most studied cannabinoids, it is not the only one with therapeutic benefits. Other cannabinoids like CBD, CBG, and CBH also have significant health benefits.

4. **"THC Is Addictive Like Hard Drugs":** THC does have a potential for dependency, but it is generally considered less addictive than many 'hard' drugs. The risk of addiction is relatively lower, and THC does not typically provoke the severe physical withdrawal symptoms seen with substances like opioids.

Addressing the Risks

To mitigate the risks associated with THC, several measures can be implemented:

1. **Education and Awareness:** Providing accurate information about the effects, risks, and safe use of THC is essential. Public education campaigns can help dispel myths and encourage responsible use.

2. **Regulation and Quality Control:** Implementing regulations to ensure the quality and safety of THC products is vital. This includes controlling the potency of THC in recreational and medical cannabis products and ensuring they are free from contaminants.

3. **Targeted Research:** Further research into the long-term effects of THC, especially on the developing brain, is necessary to better understand its risks and inform public health policies.

4. **Medical Guidance:** For medicinal users, guidance from healthcare professionals is crucial. This includes prescribing appropriate dosages, monitoring for adverse effects, and considering the patient's medical history and potential for drug interactions.

Balancing the Narrative

It is important to balance the narrative around THC by acknowledging both its benefits and risks. While THC offers significant therapeutic potential, understanding and addressing its risks ensures safer use. This balanced approach is essential for informed policy-making, medical practice, and public perception.

Future Directions

As research continues and societal attitudes evolve, the understanding of THC will become more nuanced. This will likely lead to more sophisticated methods of using THC medicinally, such as targeted therapies that minimize risks while maximizing benefits.

Additionally, evolving legal frameworks will play a crucial role in shaping the accessibility and use of THC for both medical and recreational purposes.

In conclusion, while THC is a complex and sometimes controversial compound, it holds significant medicinal value. Acknowledging and addressing the risks and misconceptions associated with THC is key to harnessing its potential responsibly. Through continued research, education, and balanced discourse, the role of THC in medicine and society can be better understood and optimized.

Chapter 3: CBD – The Wellness Warrior

CBD: Beyond the Hype

Cannabidiol (CBD), a non-psychoactive cannabinoid found in cannabis, has gained widespread popularity and interest for its potential health benefits. This section explores the reality behind the hype, examining the scientific evidence supporting CBD's therapeutic uses and its impact in various medical contexts.

Understanding CBD and Its Mechanism of Action

CBD differs significantly from THC in that it does not produce a high or psychoactive effect. Its mechanism of action is distinct; CBD interacts with the endocannabinoid system (ECS) but does so indirectly, influencing the ECS and other receptors in the body. This interaction contributes to CBD's therapeutic effects, including its anti-inflammatory, analgesic, and anxiolytic properties.

Evidence-Based Medical Benefits of CBD

1. **Epilepsy Treatment:** One of the most well-researched and proven uses of CBD is in the treatment of certain forms of epilepsy. The FDA-approved drug Epidiolex, which contains CBD, is effective in reducing the frequency of seizures in conditions like Dravet syndrome and Lennox-Gastaut syndrome.

2. **Anxiety and Depression:** CBD has shown promise in reducing symptoms of anxiety and depression. Studies suggest that CBD may alter serotonin signals, which play a role in mental health. Its potential as a treatment for anxiety disorders, PTSD, and depression is a significant area of interest.

3. **Pain and Inflammation:** CBD is widely used for its anti-inflammatory and analgesic effects. It may be beneficial in treating chronic pain, arthritis, and neuropathic pain. CBD's ability to reduce inflammation also makes it a potential therapeutic agent in autoimmune diseases and inflammatory conditions.

4. **Neuroprotective Properties:** Research is exploring CBD's role as a neuroprotective agent. It may have potential in treating neurodegenerative diseases like Alzheimer's and Parkinson's due to its ability to reduce inflammation and promote neurogenesis.

Debunking Common Misconceptions about CBD

Despite its popularity, there are several misconceptions about CBD that need to be addressed:

1. **"CBD Is a Cure-All":** While CBD has various health benefits, it is not a panacea for all illnesses. Its effects can vary, and more research is needed to understand its full potential and limitations.

2. **"All CBD Products Are the Same":** The quality and concentration of CBD can vary greatly among products. It's important for consumers to choose products from reputable sources and to be aware of the CBD content and purity.

3. **"CBD Has No Side Effects":** While generally well-tolerated, CBD can have side effects, particularly at high doses. These can include fatigue, diarrhea, and changes in appetite and weight.

Regulation and Quality Control in the CBD Industry

The rapid growth of the CBD market has outpaced regulation, leading to concerns about product quality and misleading claims. There is a need for stricter regulation and standardization to ensure the safety and efficacy of CBD products. Consumers should be cautious and seek information from reliable sources when choosing CBD products.

The Future of CBD Research and Applications

The future of CBD is promising but requires further research to fully understand its therapeutic potential and to develop standardized, effective treatments. Areas of particular interest include its use in psychiatric conditions, its potential in cancer treatment, and its role in treating other chronic diseases.

In conclusion, CBD, beyond the hype, offers significant medical benefits, particularly in treating epilepsy, anxiety, and chronic pain. While it is not a cure-all, its potential as a therapeutic agent is substantial. As research continues and the industry matures, the role of CBD in medicine is likely to expand, offering new avenues for treatment and improving the quality of life for many patients.

Therapeutic Applications of CBD

Cannabidiol (CBD), with its wide range of potential therapeutic applications, stands out as one of the most intriguing and promising compounds in modern medicine. This section delves into the various therapeutic uses of CBD, examining how it can be applied to treat different health conditions and enhance overall well-being.

CBD in Pain Management

One of the most common uses of CBD is in the management of pain. Its analgesic and anti-inflammatory properties make it a compelling alternative for treating chronic pain, including conditions like arthritis and multiple sclerosis. CBD may offer a more natural approach to pain relief, especially for those seeking alternatives to traditional painkillers that can have significant side effects.

CBD in Mental Health Treatment

CBD's potential in treating mental health conditions is a rapidly growing area of interest. Its anxiolytic properties make it a viable option for treating anxiety disorders, including generalized anxiety disorder, social anxiety disorder, and panic disorder. Furthermore, preliminary studies suggest that CBD may be beneficial in treating depression, PTSD, and even addiction, providing a novel approach to mental health care.

CBD and Neurological Disorders

Research into CBD's neuroprotective properties has opened up new possibilities for treating neurological disorders. In epilepsy, CBD has proven effective in reducing seizure frequency, leading to the development of the first FDA-approved CBD-based medication, Epidiolex. Additionally, CBD is being studied for its potential in treating other neurological conditions like Alzheimer's disease, Parkinson's disease, and stroke, due to its anti-inflammatory and antioxidant effects.

CBD in Autoimmune Diseases and Inflammation

CBD's anti-inflammatory properties are particularly relevant in the context of autoimmune diseases. It has shown promise in modulating the immune system and reducing inflammation, which can be beneficial in conditions like rheumatoid arthritis, inflammatory bowel disease, and psoriasis. By targeting inflammatory pathways, CBD offers a potential therapeutic avenue for managing these often debilitating conditions.

CBD in Oncology

The role of CBD in cancer treatment is an area of ongoing research. While not a cure for cancer, CBD may help alleviate some of the symptoms associated with cancer and its treatment, such as pain, nausea, and appetite loss. There is also growing interest in CBD's potential anti-tumor properties and its ability to enhance the efficacy of certain chemotherapy agents.

CBD for Skin Health

In dermatology, CBD is gaining attention for its potential in treating various skin conditions. Its anti-inflammatory and antioxidative properties may help in managing acne, eczema, and psoriasis.

CBD-infused skincare products are also being explored for their potential to improve skin health and appearance.

Challenges and Considerations in Using CBD Therapeutically

While the therapeutic potential of CBD is significant, there are several challenges and considerations in its use:

1. **Dosage and Administration:** Determining the optimal dosage and administration method of CBD for different conditions is a major challenge. Factors like body weight, the nature of the condition, and individual physiology can affect how CBD works.

2. **Regulatory and Legal Issues:** The legal status of CBD varies by region and is often complex. This impacts both research into CBD and its availability for therapeutic use.

3. **Quality Control and Standardization:** The CBD market is currently flooded with products of varying quality and potency. Ensuring the standardization and quality of CBD products is crucial for both safety and efficacy.

Future Directions in CBD Therapy

The future of CBD therapy is promising, with ongoing research likely to expand its therapeutic applications and refine how it is used. Clinical trials and scientific studies are crucial for establishing CBD's efficacy and safety profile for various conditions. As our understanding of CBD grows, so does the potential for developing targeted treatments that leverage its therapeutic properties.

One of the exciting prospects is the personalized medicine approach in CBD therapy. By understanding individual responses to CBD, treatments can be tailored to maximize efficacy while minimizing side effects. This approach could revolutionize how we treat a range of conditions, from chronic pain to mental health disorders.

Furthermore, the integration of CBD into complementary therapies offers another promising avenue. Using CBD in conjunction with other treatments, whether pharmacological or holistic, could enhance overall treatment effectiveness and patient well-being.

Educating Healthcare Professionals and Patients

A critical aspect of advancing CBD therapy is educating both healthcare professionals and patients. As CBD becomes more prevalent in therapeutic settings, it's essential that practitioners are knowledgeable about its uses, benefits, and risks. Similarly, educating patients on how to use CBD safely and effectively is key to maximizing its therapeutic potential.

Navigating the Legal Landscape

The evolving legal landscape surrounding CBD will also play a significant role in its future as a therapeutic agent. As regulations change and become more standardized, it's likely that access to high-quality, medically approved CBD products will increase, making it a more viable treatment option for a broader range of patients.

In conclusion, the therapeutic applications of CBD are vast and varied, offering significant potential in treating a wide array of health conditions. From pain management to mental health treatment, CBD's role in medicine continues to expand as we learn more about its capabilities. By addressing challenges in dosage, quality control, and regulation, and by continuing to invest in research and education, the full therapeutic potential of CBD can be realized, offering new hope and options for patients worldwide.

CBD in Everyday Life

Cannabidiol (CBD), once a niche compound known only in certain medical and scientific circles, has rapidly integrated into everyday life. This section explores how CBD has become a commonplace wellness supplement and its growing presence in various aspects of daily living.

The Rise of CBD in Wellness Culture

CBD's surge in popularity can largely be attributed to its perceived health benefits without the psychoactive effects associated with THC. This has made CBD an appealing option for those seeking natural alternatives for stress relief, pain management, and overall wellness. Its non-intoxicating nature means it can be incorporated into daily routines without disrupting normal activities.

CBD in Consumer Products

The market has seen an influx of CBD-infused products, ranging from dietary supplements to beauty products. These include oils, capsules, topical creams, bath bombs, and even edibles like gummies and chocolates. The versatility of CBD has allowed it to be integrated into various product forms, catering to diverse consumer preferences and needs.

CBD for Stress and Anxiety Management

One of the most common uses of CBD in everyday life is for stress and anxiety management. Many individuals turn to CBD products to help alleviate daily stressors and promote a sense of calm. While scientific evidence continues to evolve, anecdotal reports from users often cite positive effects on their mental well-being.

CBD in Skincare and Cosmetics

The skincare and cosmetic industry has embraced CBD for its potential anti-inflammatory and antioxidant properties. CBD is increasingly found in products like creams, serums, and lotions, touted for its ability to soothe skin, reduce redness, and even combat signs of aging. The appeal of natural, plant-based ingredients in skincare has further propelled CBD's popularity in this sector.

CBD for Sleep and Relaxation

Another common application of CBD in everyday life is as a sleep aid. Many users report that CBD helps them relax and improve their sleep quality. While research in this area is ongoing, the potential of CBD to aid in sleep without the side effects of traditional sleep medications is a significant draw for many.

CBD in Fitness and Recovery

Athletes and fitness enthusiasts are increasingly turning to CBD for its potential benefits in workout recovery. CBD's anti-inflammatory properties may help in reducing muscle soreness and speeding up recovery, making it a popular supplement in sports and fitness communities.

Navigating the Legal and Regulatory Aspects

Despite its widespread availability, the legal status of CBD can be complex and varies by region. Consumers need to be aware of their local laws regarding CBD use and purchase. Additionally, the lack of regulation in the CBD market means that product quality can vary significantly, underscoring the importance of choosing reputable brands and products.

The Importance of Education and Research

As CBD becomes more integrated into everyday life, education and research are crucial. Consumers should be informed about the potential benefits and limitations of CBD, as well as how to choose and use products safely. Ongoing research is essential to provide a scientific basis for CBD's use and to guide its safe and effective incorporation into daily routines.

Future Trends in CBD Use

The future of CBD in everyday life looks promising, with potential for new and innovative products and applications. As research provides deeper insights into CBD's effects and benefits, it's likely that its use will become more refined and targeted. This could lead to CBD products tailored for specific health and wellness goals, further solidifying its place in daily life.

In conclusion, CBD's integration into everyday life reflects a growing trend towards natural wellness solutions. Its versatility, non-psychoactive nature, and potential health benefits have made it a popular choice for a wide range of consumers. As the market continues to evolve and research expands our understanding of CBD, its role in daily health and wellness routines is likely to grow, offering new opportunities for natural, plant-based care in our everyday lives.

Chapter 4:
CBG – The Rising Star

CBG: An Overview

Cannabigerol (CBG), often referred to as the "mother of all canna-binoids," is a lesser-known compound in cannabis that has begun to attract significant scientific and medical interest. This section provides an overview of CBG, discussing its properties, how it differs from other cannabinoids like THC and CBD, and its potential therapeutic applications.

Understanding CBG and Its Unique Role

CBG is considered a minor cannabinoid because it is present in lower concentrations in most cannabis strains compared to THC and CBD. However, its significance lies in its role as a precursor to other cannabinoids. In the cannabis plant, CBG-A, the acidic form of CBG, is the first cannabinoid that forms. As the plant matures, CBG-A is converted into other cannabinoids, primarily THC and CBD, through enzymatic processes.

Extraction and Isolation of CBG

The lower concentration of CBG in cannabis plants presents a chal-lenge for extraction and isolation. This has historically made CBG less accessible and more expensive to produce than THC or CBD. However, advances in cultivation and extraction techniques are enabling the production of higher yields of CBG, making it more available for research and therapeutic use.

Potential Medical Benefits of CBG

Research into CBG is still in its early stages, but initial studies sug-gest it may have several therapeutic benefits:

1. **Neuroprotective Properties:** CBG has shown potential as a neuroprotectant, possibly offering benefits for neurodegenerative diseases like Huntington's disease. Early studies suggest it might help protect neurons and support brain health.

2. **Anti-Inflammatory Effects:** Like CBD, CBG appears to have anti-inflammatory properties, which could be beneficial in treating conditions like inflammatory bowel disease and Crohn's disease.

3. **Antibacterial and Antimicrobial Properties:** CBG has demonstrated antibacterial and antimicrobial effects, particularly against drug-resistant bacteria like MRSA, indicating potential use in fighting infections.

4. **Cancer Research:** Preliminary research suggests that CBG may have properties that could be useful in cancer treatment. It has been observed to block receptors that cause cancer cell growth in certain types of cancer, such as colorectal cancer, though much more research is needed in this area.

CBG vs. THC and CBD

Unlike THC, CBG does not have psychoactive properties and does not produce a high. This makes it an attractive option for medical applications where the psychoactive effects of THC are undesirable. Compared to CBD, CBG is less studied, but it may offer distinct therapeutic benefits that differ from those of CBD, particularly in its neuroprotective and antibacterial properties.

Challenges in CBG Research and Use

The primary challenges in CBG research and use are related to its availability and the cost of production. Since CBG is present in lower concentrations in cannabis plants, producing sufficient quantities for research and therapeutic use is more resource-intensive compared to THC and CBD. However, with the development of specialized strains and advanced extraction techniques, these challenges are gradually being overcome.

Regulatory Aspects of CBG

As with other cannabinoids, the legal and regulatory status of CBG varies by region. In many places, regulations are still catching up with the evolving landscape of cannabinoid research and use. As interest in CBG grows, it is likely that specific regulations concerning its production, sale, and use will be developed.

The Future of CBG

The future of CBG looks promising as research continues to uncover its potential health benefits. With ongoing advancements in cannabis cultivation and extraction technology, it is likely that CBG will become more accessible and affordable, leading to wider use in therapeutic applications.

In conclusion, CBG is an exciting and relatively unexplored cannabinoid with significant potential for a variety of medical applications. As research into CBG expands, it is poised to become an important player in the field of cannabinoid therapy, offering new possibilities for treatment and enhancing our understanding of the therapeutic potential of cannabis.

Potential Health Benefits of CBG

Cannabigerol (CBG), though less known than its counterparts THC and CBD, has started to gain attention in the scientific community for its potential health benefits. This section explores the emerging research on CBG and its possible therapeutic applications.

Neuroprotective Effects

One of the most promising areas of CBG research is its potential as a neuroprotective agent. Early studies indicate that CBG may offer benefits in neurodegenerative diseases like Huntington's disease and multiple sclerosis. Its neuroprotective properties could help in preserving nerve cells and supporting brain health, potentially slowing the progression of these diseases.

Anti-Inflammatory Properties

CBG has shown significant anti-inflammatory effects, which could be beneficial in treating a range of inflammatory conditions. It may have applications in inflammatory bowel diseases such as Crohn's disease and ulcerative colitis, offering a potential alternative to traditional treatments that often have significant side effects.

Antibacterial and Antimicrobial Properties

Remarkably, CBG has demonstrated strong antibacterial and antimicrobial properties, especially against drug-resistant bacterial strains like MRSA (Methicillin-resistant Staphylococcus aureus). This suggests that CBG could be developed into a novel antibacterial agent, addressing the growing issue of antibiotic resistance.

Cancer Treatment Potential

Preliminary research has suggested that CBG might possess anti-cancer properties. Some studies have observed CBG blocking receptors that cause cancer cell growth, particularly in colorectal cancer. Although this research is in its infancy, it opens the door to the possibility of CBG playing a role in future cancer treatments.

Appetite Stimulation

CBG has been found to stimulate appetite in animal studies. This could make it a valuable tool in treating conditions such as cachexia (wasting syndrome) often associated with chronic illnesses like cancer and HIV/AIDS. Unlike THC, which also stimulates appetite, CBG does not produce psychoactive effects, making it a more suitable option for some patients.

Glaucoma and Ocular Health

Research suggests that CBG may be beneficial for treating glaucoma by reducing intraocular pressure. Its vasodilator and neuroprotective properties could help in preserving the health of the optic nerve, offering a potential therapeutic option for this condition.

Anxiety and Depression

While CBD is more commonly associated with treating anxiety and depression, CBG also shows potential in this area. Its ability to boost anandamide, a naturally occurring cannabinoid in the brain known as the "bliss molecule," suggests that CBG could help regulate mood and offer anti-anxiety and antidepressant effects.

Pain Relief

CBG might be effective in managing pain without the psychoactive effects of THC. Its analgesic properties, combined with its ability to combat inflammation, make it a promising candidate for developing new pain relief treatments, especially for conditions that are difficult to treat with current pain medications.

Challenges and Future Research

Despite these potential health benefits, research on CBG is still in the early stages. One of the main challenges is the low concentration of CBG in most cannabis strains, which makes its extraction and isolation more difficult and expensive. However, as interest in CBG grows, cultivation techniques are evolving to produce higher yields of this cannabinoid.

Future research will need to focus on clinical trials to better understand CBG's therapeutic potential and safety profile. This will involve not only exploring its benefits for specific conditions but also understanding how it interacts with other medications and potential side effects.

Regulatory Landscape for CBG

As with other cannabinoids, the legal and regulatory landscape for CBG is complex and varies by jurisdiction. The evolving status of cannabis and hemp laws worldwide will play a significant role in determining the availability and research of CBG in the future.

Conclusion

CBG holds great promise as a therapeutic agent, with potential applications ranging from neuroprotection and cancer treatment to pain management and mental health. As the body of research grows, CBG may become a significant player in the field of cannabinoid-based therapies, offering new options for patients with various health conditions. The future of CBG in medicine is exciting, and continued research and development will be key to unlocking its full therapeutic potential.

Research and Future Prospects of CBG

Cannabigerol (CBG) is emerging as a cannabinoid with immense potential, sparking significant interest in the scientific community. This section examines the current state of CBG research and discusses the future prospects of this relatively unknown but promising cannabinoid.

Current State of CBG Research

Research on CBG is still in its nascent stages, especially when compared to its more studied counterparts, THC and CBD. However, the existing studies have shown promising results in several areas:

1. **Neuroprotection:** CBG has shown potential in protecting neurons and could be beneficial in neurodegenerative diseases like Huntington's and Parkinson's.

2. **Cancer Research:** Early studies suggest that CBG may inhibit the growth of certain cancer cells, indicating potential use in cancer therapy.

3. **Anti-Inflammatory and Analgesic Properties:** CBG's effectiveness in reducing inflammation and pain points to its potential in treating conditions like inflammatory bowel disease and chronic pain.

4. **Antibacterial Properties:** CBG's ability to combat bacterial strains, including MRSA, is particularly notable given the increasing antibiotic resistance.

Despite these promising findings, most of the current research on CBG is limited to preclinical studies, primarily in vitro and animal models. There is a significant need for clinical trials to fully understand CBG's therapeutic potential and safety in humans.

Challenges in CBG Research

One of the primary challenges in CBG research is the cannabinoid's low concentration in cannabis plants, making it less economically viable to extract and study compared to THC and CBD. However, the development of specialized cannabis strains with higher CBG content and advances in extraction technology are beginning to mitigate this challenge.

Another issue is the regulatory landscape surrounding cannabis and cannabinoids, which can vary significantly between regions and often limits research opportunities.

Future Prospects and Areas of Interest

The future of CBG research looks promising, with several key areas of interest:

1. **Neurological Disorders:** Given its neuroprotective properties, further research into CBG's potential in treating neurological conditions is highly anticipated.

2. **Oncology:** The exploration of CBG's anti-cancer properties is an exciting area, with the potential for CBG to complement existing cancer treatments.

3. **Antimicrobial Uses:** As antibiotic resistance becomes a global health concern, CBG's efficacy against resistant bacterial strains could lead to new types of antibiotics.

4. **Chronic Pain and Inflammation:** CBG's role in pain and inflammation management could provide new treatment options for chronic pain conditions, offering an alternative to opioids and other pain relievers with significant side effects.

5. **Mental Health:** Research into CBG's effects on anxiety and mood disorders could expand the options available for mental health treatment.

The Role of Genetics and Cultivation in CBG Production

Advancements in genetic engineering and cultivation techniques play a crucial role in the future of CBG research. By developing cannabis strains that yield higher concentrations of CBG, researchers can more efficiently study the compound and explore its therapeutic potential. Genetic manipulation of the cannabis plant may also lead to the discovery of new cannabinoids with unique health benefits.

Potential for Personalized Medicine

CBG's diverse therapeutic potential opens up possibilities for personalized medicine. As research advances, CBG could be tailored to individual needs, offering targeted treatments based on specific medical conditions and patient profiles. This personalized approach could revolutionize how we approach cannabinoid therapy, maximizing benefits while minimizing side effects.

Integrating CBG into Mainstream Medicine

For CBG to become a part of mainstream medicine, there needs to be a concerted effort in clinical trials and regulatory approvals. This includes understanding the appropriate dosages, delivery methods, and long-term effects of CBG use. Establishing clear guidelines and ensuring product consistency and quality will be crucial for its integration into healthcare practices.

Educational Initiatives and Public Awareness

As CBG gains prominence, educating healthcare professionals and the public about its benefits and limitations is vital. Dispelling myths and providing evidence-based information will be key to its acceptance and safe use.

Collaboration Between Researchers and Industry

The future of CBG research also depends on collaboration between academic researchers, medical professionals, and the cannabis industry. Such partnerships can facilitate the development of high-quality CBG products and ensure that research is translated into practical, therapeutic applications.

Potential Economic Impact

The growing interest in CBG could also have significant economic implications. As demand increases, the cultivation and production of CBG-rich cannabis strains could become a lucrative sector within the cannabis industry, encouraging further investment in research and development.

Conclusion

The research and future prospects of CBG are marked by both challenges and opportunities. Its potential as a therapeutic agent is vast, with possibilities ranging from treating neurological disorders to combating antibiotic-resistant bacteria. As research progresses, CBG could become an essential component of cannabinoid-based therapies, offering new hope for patients with a variety of health conditions. The key to unlocking CBG's full potential lies in continued research, collaboration, and innovation, paving the way for its integration into modern medicine.

Chapter 5:
CBH – The New Frontier

Discovering CBH

Cannabihexol (CBH) is one of the newest cannabinoids to be identified, adding to the ever-expanding list of compounds found in the cannabis plant. This section explores the discovery of CBH, what sets it apart from other cannabinoids, and the potential implications of this discovery for medical science and the cannabis industry.

The Discovery of CBH

CBH was identified relatively recently in comparison to more well-known cannabinoids like THC and CBD. Its discovery was a result of advanced analytical techniques and a deeper exploration of the cannabis plant's complex chemistry. CBH is found in very low concentrations in the plant, making it a rare and less-studied cannabinoid.

Chemical Structure and Properties

The chemical structure of CBH is unique and differs from other cannabinoids, which hints at potentially different interactions with the human body's endocannabinoid system (ECS). This unique structure raises questions about how CBH might affect the body and whether it has distinct properties or health benefits compared to other cannabinoids.

Early Research and Potential Benefits

Research on CBH is still in its infancy, but initial studies and interest suggest that it may have unique benefits or applications. Given the diversity of effects seen with other cannabinoids, researchers are keen to explore the full spectrum of CBH's potential, from its therapeutic properties to its impact on physiology.

Challenges in Studying CBH

The primary challenge in studying CBH is its rarity in the cannabis plant. This scarcity makes extraction and study more difficult and costly compared to other, more abundant cannabinoids. Advances in cultivation and extraction technology will be key to facilitating more comprehensive research on CBH.

CBH's Interaction with the ECS

Understanding how CBH interacts with the ECS is crucial. The ECS plays a vital role in regulating various bodily functions, and each cannabinoid can affect this system differently. Investigating CBH's interaction with ECS receptors could provide insights into its potential therapeutic applications and help differentiate it from other cannabinoids.

Potential Medical Applications

Given the therapeutic benefits of other cannabinoids, there is significant interest in exploring similar possibilities for CBH. It may have potential in treating specific medical conditions, contributing to pain management, reducing inflammation, or offering neuroprotective effects, among other applications.

Comparative Studies with Other Cannabinoids

Comparing CBH with other cannabinoids like THC, CBD, and CBG can offer valuable insights. These comparative studies could reveal unique properties of CBH, leading to targeted applications in cannabinoid-based therapies.

The Role of Technology in CBH Research

Advancements in technology, particularly in the fields of genetics and extraction, are pivotal in exploring CBH. These technologies could enable the production of cannabis strains with higher concentrations of CBH or more efficient extraction methods, making research more feasible.

Regulatory and Legal Considerations

As with other cannabinoids, the legal and regulatory landscape will influence the study and use of CBH. Understanding and navigating these regulations is essential for advancing research and potential medical applications.

Future Prospects in CBH Research

The future of CBH research holds promise but requires a focused effort to understand its properties and potential benefits. As interest in the medical potential of cannabinoids continues to grow, CBH could become an important subject of study and a valuable addition to cannabinoid therapies.

Educational and Awareness Efforts

Educating the medical community and the public about CBH and its potential is important. As research progresses, disseminating accurate and evidence-based information will be crucial in shaping the perception and use of CBH.

Conclusion

The discovery of CBH adds a new dimension to the world of cannabinoids and their potential applications. While still at a very early stage of research, CBH presents an intriguing opportunity for medical science and the cannabis industry. Continued research, technological advancements, and a supportive regulatory environment will be key to unlocking the mysteries of CBH and harnessing its possible benefits.

Current Studies and Findings on CBH

Cannabihexol (CBH), as one of the newest cannabinoids to be discovered, presents an exciting frontier in cannabinoid research. This section delves into the current studies and findings on CBH, discussing what is known so far and the potential implications of these early discoveries.

The Rarity and Novelty of CBH

CBH's rarity in the cannabis plant has made it a subject of intrigue in the scientific community. Its recent discovery means that research is still very much in the preliminary stages, but the interest it has generated is significant. The novelty of CBH lies in its unique chemical structure, which suggests it may interact with the body's endocannabinoid system (ECS) differently from better-known cannabinoids like THC and CBD.

Initial Research Focus

The initial research on CBH has primarily focused on understanding its basic properties and how it differs from other cannabinoids. These early studies are crucial for laying the groundwork for more detailed investigations into CBH's potential therapeutic effects.

Potential Therapeutic Effects

Although research is in its early stages, there is speculation that CBH could possess unique therapeutic effects. Given the varied medical applications of other cannabinoids, scientists are exploring whether CBH could offer new treatment possibilities, particularly in areas where current cannabinoid therapies may fall short.

CBH and the Endocannabinoid System

One key area of research is understanding how CBH interacts with the ECS. The ECS plays a critical role in regulating a wide range of physiological processes, and each cannabinoid has a unique way of influencing this system. Early indications suggest that CBH might bind to ECS receptors differently than THC or CBD, which could result in distinct effects on the body.

Comparisons with Other Cannabinoids

Comparative studies are being planned to contrast CBH with other cannabinoids. These comparisons are important for identifying any unique properties or advantages that CBH might have. For example, if CBH is found to have stronger anti-inflammatory or neuroprotective effects than its counterparts, it could open up new avenues in the treatment of certain conditions.

Challenges in CBH Research

The primary challenge in studying CBH is its low natural occurrence in cannabis plants, making it difficult and expensive to extract in significant quantities. This scarcity poses a barrier to extensive research and clinical trials, which are necessary to fully understand and validate CBH's therapeutic potential.

Technological Advances in CBH Extraction

Advances in extraction technology and the development of specialized cannabis strains could help overcome these challenges. There is growing interest in genetic modification and selective breeding techniques to increase the yield of CBH in cannabis plants, facilitating more accessible and cost-effective research.

Regulatory Landscape for CBH Research

The legal and regulatory framework surrounding cannabis and cannabinoids impacts the ability to conduct comprehensive CBH research. Navigating these regulations, which can vary significantly across different regions, is a crucial aspect of advancing studies on CBH. As interest in CBH grows, it may prompt changes in regulations to support more extensive research.

Clinical Trials and Human Studies

The next step in CBH research involves clinical trials and human studies, which are essential to determine its efficacy and safety. These studies will provide valuable insights into how CBH can be used therapeutically, including potential dosages, delivery methods, and target conditions.

Exploring Synergistic Effects with Other Cannabinoids

Another interesting area of research is exploring the synergistic effects of CBH when combined with other cannabinoids. This could lead to the development of new cannabinoid-based therapies that leverage the combined benefits of multiple compounds for enhanced therapeutic effects.

Potential Applications in Medicine

Based on the properties of other cannabinoids, CBH could have applications in various medical areas, such as pain management, inflammation control, neuroprotection, and possibly even in the treatment of certain mental health conditions. However, these potential applications remain speculative until more research is conducted.

Educational Efforts and Public Awareness

As research on CBH progresses, it will be important to educate both the medical community and the general public about its findings. Dispelling myths and providing accurate information will be crucial in shaping the understanding and potential use of CBH in healthcare.

Conclusion

Current studies and findings on CBH represent just the beginning of what could be a significant new chapter in cannabinoid research. While much remains to be discovered, the early interest in CBH underscores the potential for new therapeutic applications and a deeper understanding of the endocannabinoid system. Continued research, supported by advancements in technology and an evolving regulatory landscape, will be key to unlocking the full potential of this intriguing new cannabinoid.

The Potential Impact of CBH in Medicine

Cannabihexol (CBH), as one of the latest cannabinoids to be discovered, presents an intriguing potential in the realm of medical science. This section explores the potential impact of CBH in medicine, considering its unique properties and how it might contribute to future treatments and healthcare practices.

Unique Properties of CBH

CBH stands out due to its rarity and distinctive chemical structure, suggesting it may have different effects compared to more well-known cannabinoids like THC and CBD. Understanding these unique properties is crucial, as it could lead to the discovery of new mechanisms for treating diseases or managing symptoms.

Potential Therapeutic Applications

While research is still in the early stages, the potential therapeutic applications of CBH are promising. Its distinct interaction with the endocannabinoid system (ECS) may offer new ways to target various health conditions, potentially including:

1. **Neurodegenerative Diseases:** Given the neuroprotective properties observed in other cannabinoids, CBH could play a role in treating conditions like Alzheimer's and Parkinson's disease.

2. **Inflammatory Conditions:** If CBH possesses anti-inflammatory properties, it could be useful in treating inflammatory diseases such as rheumatoid arthritis or Crohn's disease.

3. **Pain Management:** CBH might offer an alternative approach to pain relief, particularly for chronic pain conditions, without the psychoactive effects of THC.

4. **Cancer Therapy:** Like other cannabinoids, CBH could potentially be used in cancer treatment, either to alleviate symptoms or possibly as an anti-tumor agent.

Advancing Research and Clinical Trials

The full potential of CBH in medicine can only be realized through comprehensive research and clinical trials. These studies are essential to determine the efficacy, safety, and optimal use of CBH in various medical contexts. Clinical trials will provide the much-needed data to understand how CBH interacts with the human body and its possible side effects.

Potential for Personalized Medicine

CBH could contribute to the field of personalized medicine, where treatments are tailored to individual patient needs. By understanding how different people respond to CBH, it could be used to develop personalized treatment plans, enhancing the effectiveness and reducing the risk of adverse effects.

Challenges in CBH Research and Development

One of the main challenges in realizing the medical potential of CBH is its rarity in cannabis plants. Overcoming this requires advancements in cultivation and extraction techniques. Additionally, navigating the complex regulatory landscape of cannabinoids is crucial for facilitating research and application in medical settings.

Educational and Ethical Considerations

As with any new medical treatment, educating healthcare providers and patients about CBH is vital. This includes understanding its uses, potential benefits, and risks. Ethical considerations, particularly in terms of accessibility and fair distribution, will also play a crucial role as CBH potentially enters mainstream medicine.

Integrating CBH into Existing Treatment Regimens

Exploring how CBH can be integrated into existing treatment regimens is another important aspect. This involves understanding how it interacts with other medications and how it can complement conventional treatments to provide holistic care.

Global Health Implications

The discovery of CBH and its potential application in medicine could have global health implications. In regions where access to certain medications is limited, CBH could offer an alternative treatment option. However, ensuring global access and addressing disparities in healthcare will be key challenges.

The Future of CBH in Medicine

The future of CBH in medicine is full of possibilities but hinges on continued research and development. As we deepen our understanding of this cannabinoid, its role in treating various health conditions could become more significant. CBH may also inspire further exploration into other lesser-known cannabinoids, broadening the horizons of cannabinoid-based medicine.

Collaboration Between Researchers, Clinicians, and Industry

Effective collaboration between researchers, clinicians, and the cannabis industry will be crucial for advancing CBH's medical applications. This collaboration can accelerate the translation of research findings into practical treatments and ensure that innovations in CBH therapy are grounded in scientific evidence.

Regulatory Evolution and Standardization

The evolution of regulatory frameworks will significantly impact the medical use of CBH. Establishing standardized guidelines for the production, quality control, and prescription of CBH-based treatments will be essential for patient safety and efficacy.

Public Perception and Acceptance

The public's perception of cannabinoids and their acceptance in medical treatment can influence the adoption of CBH-based therapies. Continued efforts to educate the public and dispel myths about cannabinoids are necessary to foster a supportive environment for CBH's medical use.

Conclusion

The potential impact of CBH in medicine is a compelling subject that stands at the intersection of scientific discovery and health-care innovation. While there are challenges to overcome, the possibilities for CBH to contribute to medical science and patient care are significant. Continued research, collaboration, and open-mindedness will be key to unlocking the full therapeutic potential of this intriguing cannabinoid, potentially leading to groundbreaking advancements in medical treatments.

Chapter 6: Synergistic Effects and the Entourage Effect

Understanding the Entourage Effect

The concept of the entourage effect is a pivotal aspect of cannabinoid science, proposing that cannabinoids such as THC, CBD, CBG, and CBH work more effectively when used together rather than in isolation. This section explores the entourage effect, its implications in medical applications, and how it shapes our understanding of cannabinoid therapies.

The Basis of the Entourage Effect

The entourage effect is based on the premise that the various components of the cannabis plant, including cannabinoids, terpenes, and flavonoids, interact synergistically to enhance each other's effects. This synergy potentially amplifies the therapeutic benefits and mitigates the side effects of individual cannabinoids.

Evidence Supporting the Entourage Effect

While the entourage effect is widely accepted in the cannabis community, scientific evidence Is still emerging. Some studies have shown that whole-plant extracts, containing a spectrum of cannabinoids and other compounds, are more effective or have fewer side effects than isolated cannabinoids. This suggests that the compounds in cannabis may work together in a way that maximizes therapeutic potential.

Implications for Medical Cannabis Use

The entourage effect has significant implications for medical cannabis use. It suggests that full-spectrum cannabis extracts, which contain a variety of cannabinoids and other plant compounds, may be more effective than products containing a single isolated cannabinoid. This could influence the development of cannabinoid-based medications and the prescription practices of medical professionals.

Customizing Cannabinoid Therapies

Understanding the entourage effect can lead to more personalized and effective cannabinoid therapies. By tailoring the cannabinoid and terpene profiles in cannabis products, treatments can be customized to target specific symptoms or conditions more effectively.

Research Challenges and Considerations

Researching the entourage effect presents unique challenges. The complexity of cannabis chemistry, with its hundreds of potentially bioactive compounds, makes it difficult to pinpoint exactly how these components interact. Additionally, individual variability in response to cannabinoid therapies adds another layer of complexity to studying and validating the entourage effect.

Potential for New Treatment Discoveries

Exploring the entourage effect opens up possibilities for new treatment discoveries. As researchers gain a deeper understanding of how different cannabinoids and terpenes interact, they could develop novel therapies that harness these synergistic effects for specific medical conditions.

Regulatory Impacts on Research and Use

The legal and regulatory landscape significantly impacts the ability to research and utilize the entourage effect in medical treatments. In regions with restrictive cannabis laws, studying the full spectrum of cannabis compounds can be challenging, limiting the development of entourage-based therapies.

Educational Needs and Misconceptions

There is a need for education around the entourage effect, both within the medical community and among patients. Dispelling misconceptions and providing evidence-based information is crucial for the proper understanding and application of entourage-based therapies.

Future Directions in Entourage Effect Research

Future research into the entourage effect should focus on clinical trials and detailed pharmacological studies. These studies could provide clearer evidence of the entourage effect and help identify the most effective combinations of cannabinoids and terpenes for various medical applications.

Conclusion

The concept of the entourage effect represents a fascinating and potentially transformative aspect of cannabinoid science. It challenges the traditional approach of isolating active ingredients and highlights the complexity and potential of plant-based medicine. Understanding and harnessing the entourage effect could lead to more effective and personalized medical treatments, offering new hope for patients with a variety of conditions. Continued research, collaboration, and an open-minded approach to cannabis science will be key to unlocking the full potential of the entourage effect in medicine.

Synergy Among THC, CBD, CBG, and CBH

The interplay and synergy among various cannabinoids, particularly THC, CBD, CBG, and CBH, form a crucial aspect of the entourage effect and its application in medical science. This section delves into the synergistic relationships among these cannabinoids and how they might enhance each other's therapeutic effects.

THC and CBD: Complementary Interactions

One of the most researched synergies in the cannabinoid world is that between THC and CBD. THC, known for its psychoactive properties, and CBD, famous for its non-psychoactive effects, have been found to work in tandem in various therapeutic contexts. CBD is known to mitigate some of the less desirable effects of THC, such as anxiety and paranoia, while enhancing its pain-relieving properties. This complementary interaction suggests a balanced approach to using these cannabinoids can yield more effective results in treatments.

CBG and Its Role in Synergy

CBG, though less studied, is emerging as a crucial player in the cannabinoid synergy. Its ability to act as a precursor to THC and CBD, as well as its own unique properties, makes it a valuable component in cannabinoid-based therapies. CBG's potential neuroprotective and anti-inflammatory effects could enhance the therapeutic effects of both THC and CBD, especially in treating conditions like neurodegenerative diseases and inflammatory disorders.

CBH: The New Frontier in Cannabinoid Synergy

CBH, the newest cannabinoid on the block, adds another layer to the potential synergistic relationships. While research is still in its early stages, CBH could offer unique benefits that complement those of THC, CBD, and CBG. Understanding how CBH interacts with these other cannabinoids could lead to the development of more comprehensive and effective cannabinoid-based treatments.

Potential Therapeutic Combinations

Exploring different combinations of THC, CBD, CBG, and CBH can lead to optimized treatments for various medical conditions. For instance, a combination that includes CBD might be more suitable for anxiety disorders due to its anxiolytic properties, while a combination leaning more towards CBG and CBH might be better for inflammatory diseases.

Clinical Research and Trials

To fully understand and utilize the synergy among these cannabinoids, clinical research and trials are essential. These studies could help determine the most effective combinations and ratios for treating specific conditions, taking into account factors such as efficacy, safety, and side effects.

Challenges in Researching Cannabinoid Synergy

One of the main challenges in researching the synergy among THC, CBD, CBG, and CBH is the complex nature of cannabis pharmacology. Each cannabinoid has multiple mechanisms of action, and their interactions can vary based on concentration, the presence of other compounds, and individual patient factors.

Personalized Medicine and Cannabinoid Synergy

The concept of personalized medicine is particularly relevant when considering cannabinoid synergy. Individual responses to cannabinoids can vary significantly, so understanding these synergistic relationships can lead to more personalized and effective treatment plans. Tailoring cannabinoid combinations and dosages to individual patient needs could significantly enhance treatment outcomes.

Regulatory Considerations and Standardization

Navigating the regulatory landscape is crucial for advancing research into cannabinoid synergy. Standardizing cannabinoid profiles in medical products can ensure consistency and safety for patients. This standardization is particularly important when combining cannabinoids like THC, which is psychoactive, with non-psychoactive compounds like CBD, CBG, and CBH.

The Future of Cannabinoid Synergy in Medicine

The future of cannabinoid synergy in medicine looks promising. As research continues to evolve, it could lead to a new generation of cannabinoid-based therapies that are more effective and have fewer side effects than current treatments. This could revolutionize the treatment of a wide range of conditions, from chronic pain and inflammation to mental health disorders and neurodegenerative diseases.

Educational Efforts and Public Awareness

As the medical community embraces the potential of cannabinoid synergy, educating healthcare professionals and the public becomes increasingly important. Understanding the science behind cannabinoid interactions will be crucial for both prescribing these compounds and for patient compliance and satisfaction.

Conclusion

The synergy among THC, CBD, CBG, and CBH represents a fascinating and promising area of cannabinoid research. By harnessing the unique properties of each cannabinoid and exploring their combined effects, medical science can unlock new possibilities for treatments. Continued research, collaboration, and an informed approach will be key to fully realizing the potential of these synergistic relationships in medical applications.

Real-World Implications and Case Studies

The exploration of cannabinoids, particularly THC, CBD, CBG, and CBH, is not just confined to laboratories and theoretical models; it has significant real-world implications. This essay examines how the potential benefits of these cannabinoids are translating into practical applications and the impact they are having on individuals' lives through case studies.

Case Studies in Medical Treatment

1. **Epilepsy and CBD:** One of the most notable real-world applications of cannabinoids is the use of CBD in treating certain forms of epilepsy. The FDA approval of Epidiolex, a CBD-based medication, marked a significant milestone. Case studies have shown remarkable reductions in seizure frequency in patients with Dravet syndrome and Lennox-Gastaut syn-

drome, providing a new lease on life for many who suffered from these debilitating conditions.

2. **Chronic Pain and THC:** Numerous patients have turned to THC-based treatments for chronic pain relief, where conventional medications were ineffective or caused adverse side effects. Case studies illustrate how THC can improve quality of life by managing pain, enhancing sleep, and reducing reliance on opioids.

3. **CBG and Inflammatory Bowel Disease:** Although research is still emerging, there are promising reports of CBG's efficacy in treating conditions like inflammatory bowel disease. Patients who have used CBG-rich products have reported significant relief from symptoms, suggesting a potential new avenue for treatment.

CBH: Emerging Case Studies

As the newest cannabinoid under investigation, real-world applications of CBH are still in their infancy. However, early research and anecdotal evidence point to its potential in treating certain conditions, and ongoing studies are likely to provide more concrete case studies in the near future.

Cannabinoids in Mental Health

Case studies have also highlighted the role of cannabinoids in treating mental health issues like anxiety, PTSD, and depression. Patients using CBD and THC, either alone or in combination, have reported improvements in symptoms, suggesting cannabinoids could complement traditional mental health treatments.

Impact on Quality of Life

Beyond specific health conditions, cannabinoids are increasingly being recognized for their overall impact on quality of life. Patients with various chronic conditions have reported improved sleep, reduced anxiety, and a general sense of well-being after incorporating cannabinoids into their treatment regimen.

Challenges and Considerations

The real-world application of cannabinoids also brings challenges and considerations. These include ensuring consistent and standardized dosing, navigating the legal and regulatory landscape, and addressing the stigma associated with cannabis use, especially for THC.

Patient Education and Safety

Educating patients about the safe and effective use of cannabinoids is crucial. This includes understanding dosages, potential side effects, and interactions with other medications. Patient education is key to maximizing the benefits and minimizing the risks associated with cannabinoid use.

Integrating Cannabinoids into Mainstream Medicine

Integrating cannabinoids into mainstream medicine requires collaboration among healthcare providers, researchers, and policymakers. Case studies play a vital role in this process, providing tangible evidence of the benefits and challenges of cannabinoid therapies.

Future Directions and Potential

The future of cannabinoid use in medicine looks promising, with ongoing research likely to uncover more applications and refine existing treatments. As more real-world data becomes available, the full potential of cannabinoids in improving health and quality of life will become increasingly clear.

Global Health Implications

The implications of cannabinoids extend beyond individual cases to global health. As awareness grows, cannabinoids could become a crucial part of healthcare systems worldwide, offering alternative treatments for a range of conditions, especially in areas where traditional treatments are inaccessible or ineffective.

Long-Term Studies and Monitoring

Long-term studies and continued monitoring of patients using cannabinoid therapies are essential. These studies will provide valuable insights into the long-term efficacy and safety of cannabinoids, helping to guide future treatments and inform best practices.

Case Studies as a Catalyst for Change

Real-world case studies can act as a catalyst for change in the perception and acceptance of cannabinoids in medicine. They provide concrete examples of how these compounds can positively impact lives, helping to shift public and professional opinions and encouraging further research and acceptance.

Conclusion

The real-world implications and case studies of cannabinoids like THC, CBD, CBG, and CBH are a testament to their potential in transforming medical treatments and enhancing patient outcomes. As research continues to evolve, these case studies will become increasingly important in understanding the full scope of cannabinoids' impact on health and well-being. They not only highlight the therapeutic potential of these compounds but also pave the way for a more inclusive and innovative approach to healthcare.

Chapter 7: Future Directions and Challenges

The Future of Cannabinoid Research

The realm of cannabinoid research, encompassing compounds like THC, CBD, CBG, and CBH, is rapidly evolving. This section explores the potential future directions of this research, the challenges that lie ahead, and the impact it could have on medicine and science.

Advancements in Cannabinoid Science

The future of cannabinoid research promises significant advancements in our understanding of these compounds. With the discovery of new cannabinoids like CBH and ongoing studies into the properties of THC, CBD, and CBG, we are likely to see a deeper comprehension of their mechanisms of action and potential therapeutic applications.

Personalized Medicine and Cannabinoids

One of the most exciting prospects is the integration of cannabinoids into personalized medicine. Future research could lead to treatments tailored to individual genetic profiles, enhancing efficacy and reducing side effects. This personalized approach could revolutionize how we treat a range of conditions, from chronic pain to mental health disorders.

Technological Innovations in Research

Technological advancements will play a crucial role in the future of cannabinoid research. From improved extraction methods to advanced analytical tools, technology will enable researchers to study cannabinoids more effectively and uncover new aspects of their therapeutic potential.

Overcoming Research Challenges

Despite the promise, significant challenges remain in cannabinoid research. These include navigating complex regulatory environments, ensuring consistent and standardized dosing in studies, and overcoming public misconceptions about cannabinoids, particularly THC.

Expanding Clinical Trials

The expansion of clinical trials is critical for the future of cannabinoid research. These trials will provide essential data on the safety and efficacy of cannabinoids in treating various medical conditions. They will also help to clarify optimal dosages and treatment protocols.

Exploring Cannabinoid Synergy

Future research will likely delve deeper into the concept of the entourage effect and the synergy among different cannabinoids. Understanding how cannabinoids like THC, CBD, CBG, and CBH work together could lead to more effective combination therapies for a variety of health issues.

Global Health Implications

The future of cannabinoid research has significant global health implications. As knowledge about cannabinoids expands, they could become key components in global health strategies, providing alternative treatment options for diverse populations and contributing to overall health and wellness.

Ethical and Legal Considerations

As cannabinoid research advances, ethical and legal considerations will become increasingly important. This includes addressing issues related to access, affordability, and the ethical implications of using genetically modified organisms (GMOs) in cannabis cultivation.

Educational Efforts

Enhancing education around cannabinoids will be crucial in the future. This involves educating healthcare professionals, patients, and the public about the benefits, risks, and potential applications of cannabinoids in medicine.

Potential for New Therapeutic Discoveries

The ongoing exploration of cannabinoids holds the potential for new therapeutic discoveries. As researchers uncover more about cannabinoids' effects on various diseases and conditions, they could develop novel treatments that were previously unattainable.

Collaboration Across Disciplines

Future cannabinoid research will benefit from interdisciplinary collaboration. Combining insights from fields like pharmacology, genetics, neurology, and psychology can provide a more comprehensive understanding of cannabinoids and their effects on human health.

Navigating Regulatory Changes

Regulatory changes will continue to influence the trajectory of cannabinoid research. As laws and policies evolve, researchers will have greater opportunities to explore the full potential of cannabinoids, leading to more advanced and widespread applications in medicine.

Impact on Public Health Policies

The findings from future cannabinoid research could significantly impact public health policies and practices. By providing evidence-based insights into the efficacy and safety of cannabinoids, research can guide policy decisions, potentially leading to broader acceptance and integration of cannabinoid-based treatments in healthcare systems.

Sustainable and Ethical Cultivation Practices

As demand for cannabinoids increases, sustainable and ethical cultivation practices will become crucial. Future research should also focus on the environmental impact of cannabinoid production, ensuring that the growth of this field does not adversely affect the planet.

Interactions with Other Medications and Treatments

An important area of future research will be understanding how cannabinoids interact with other medications and treatments. This knowledge is essential for safely integrating cannabinoid therapies into existing treatment regimens, particularly for patients with complex medical needs.

Conclusion

The future of cannabinoid research is poised to open new frontiers in medical science and therapeutic treatments. Through continued exploration and innovation, cannabinoids like THC, CBD, CBG, and CBH could significantly transform our approach to health and wellness, offering new hope and solutions for patients worldwide. The key to this future lies in ongoing research, interdisciplinary collaboration, and a commitment to understanding the full spectrum of cannabinoids' potential.

Navigating Legal and Ethical Issues in Cannabinoid Research and Use

The evolving landscape of cannabinoid research and use, particularly concerning compounds like THC, CBD, CBG, and CBH, is rife with legal and ethical complexities. This section explores the challenges and considerations in navigating these issues, which are crucial for the responsible advancement of cannabinoid science and therapy.

The Legal Status of Cannabinoids

The legal status of cannabinoids varies widely across different regions and jurisdictions. While some countries have legalized or decriminalized cannabis and its derivatives for medical or even recreational use, others maintain strict prohibitions. This legal variability poses significant challenges for research, development, and accessibility of cannabinoid-based treatments.

Regulatory Challenges in Research

Regulatory hurdles are a major obstacle in cannabinoid research. In regions where cannabis is classified as a controlled substance, researchers face difficulties in obtaining licenses, sourcing high-quality materials, and conducting comprehensive studies. These challenges can stifle innovation and delay the development of new treatments.

Ethical Considerations in Clinical Trials

Conducting clinical trials with cannabinoids raises several ethical considerations. Ensuring informed consent, particularly in studies involving psychoactive cannabinoids like THC, is paramount. Researchers must also address potential biases and ensure that trials are designed to genuinely assess efficacy and safety.

Access and Equity in Cannabinoid Therapy

Access to cannabinoid therapies is an issue of growing concern. There is a risk that these treatments could become available only to certain segments of the population, widening health disparities. Ensuring equitable access to cannabinoid-based medicines is an ethical imperative.

Patient Safety and Public Health

Patient safety and public health considerations are central to the legal and ethical discourse on cannabinoids. Regulations governing the production, distribution, and prescription of cannabinoid products are essential to ensure patient safety and prevent misuse.

Advertising and Misinformation

The marketing of cannabinoid products, especially in regions where regulations are lax, can lead to misinformation and unrealistic expectations. Ethical marketing practices and accurate, evidence-based information are crucial to guide consumer choices and perceptions.

The Role of Healthcare Professionals

Healthcare professionals play a critical role in navigating the legal and ethical landscape of cannabinoid use. They must stay informed about the evolving legal status, clinical evidence, and best practices for prescribing cannabinoid therapies, all while adhering to ethical standards of patient care.

Intellectual Property and Commercialization

The commercialization of cannabinoid research, including patents and intellectual property rights, raises ethical questions. Balancing commercial interests with public health needs is essential to ensure that cannabinoid therapies are developed and distributed in a manner that serves the greater good.

Advocacy and Policy Influence

Advocacy groups and researchers can influence policy regarding cannabinoids. Engaging in constructive dialogue with policymakers, providing evidence-based recommendations, and advocating for responsible legal changes are crucial for advancing cannabinoid science and therapy.

Considerations in Global Health Contexts

The legal and ethical issues surrounding cannabinoids also have a global dimension. Different cultural, legal, and socio-economic contexts must be considered when advocating for policy changes or implementing cannabinoid-based therapies in diverse global health settings.

Data Privacy and Research Ethics

In cannabinoid research, particularly studies involving patient data, maintaining privacy and adhering to ethical research standards is paramount. Researchers must navigate data protection laws and ensure the confidentiality and security of participant information, especially in studies that may involve sensitive personal health data.

Balancing Risks and Benefits

Navigating the legal and ethical issues in cannabinoid research and use involves balancing the potential risks and benefits. This includes considering the implications of long-term use, the potential for dependence or misuse, and the impact of cannabinoids on different population groups, such as adolescents or individuals with mental health disorders.

Ethical Sourcing and Sustainability

Ethical sourcing and sustainability in the production of cannabinoids are emerging concerns. As demand for these compounds grows, it is crucial to ensure that their cultivation and extraction are environmentally sustainable and socially responsible.

Future Legal and Ethical Developments

The legal and ethical landscape of cannabinoid research and use is continuously evolving. Keeping abreast of these changes and anticipating future developments is essential for researchers, healthcare providers, and policymakers. This proactive approach will help ensure that cannabinoid therapies are developed and used in a manner that is legally compliant, ethically sound, and beneficial to patients.

Conclusion

Navigating the legal and ethical issues surrounding cannabinoids is a complex but essential task. It requires a multifaceted approach, involving collaboration among researchers, healthcare professionals, policymakers, and patient advocacy groups. By addressing these challenges head-on, the field of cannabinoid research and therapy can progress in a way that is responsible, equitable, and ultimately transformative for patient care.

Emerging Trends in Cannabinoid Use

The landscape of cannabinoid use, encompassing compounds such as THC, CBD, CBG, and CBH, is continually evolving. This section explores the emerging trends in cannabinoid use, both in medical contexts and broader societal applications, highlighting the shifts in perception, technology, and regulation that are shaping the future of cannabinoids.

Personalized Cannabinoid Therapies

One of the significant emerging trends is the move towards personalized cannabinoid therapies. Advances in genetics and pharmacology are enabling more tailored approaches to cannabinoid treatment, matching specific cannabinoid profiles and dosages to individual patient needs and conditions.

Innovations in Delivery Methods

Innovations in delivery methods for cannabinoids are expanding their use and effectiveness. Beyond traditional smoking or oral consumption, there are now a variety of methods including transdermal patches, nasal sprays, and even 3D-printed cannabinoid products, offering more controlled dosing and targeted delivery.

Mainstream Acceptance and Wellness Use

Cannabinoids, particularly CBD, are becoming increasingly mainstream in wellness and lifestyle products. This trend reflects a broader acceptance and recognition of the potential benefits of cannabinoids for general well-being, stress relief, and non-medical use.

Cannabinoids in Mental Health Care

There is a growing trend of using cannabinoids, particularly CBD and THC, in mental health care. Research and anecdotal evidence suggest potential benefits in treating conditions such as anxiety, depression, and PTSD, leading to increased interest from both patients and healthcare providers.

Technological Advances in Cannabinoid Production and Extraction

Technological advancements are revolutionizing the production and extraction of cannabinoids. Techniques such as CO2 extraction, molecular isolation, and biosynthesis in labs are making cannabinoid production more efficient, sustainable, and capable of yielding purer, more specific cannabinoid profiles.

Increasing Research on Lesser-Known Cannabinoids

There is a surge in research focusing on lesser-known cannabinoids like CBG and CBH. As the therapeutic potential of these cannabinoids becomes more apparent, they are likely to play a more significant role in both medical treatments and consumer products.

Regulatory Shifts and Legalization Movements

Globally, there are significant regulatory shifts and legalization movements regarding cannabis and cannabinoids. These changes are facilitating easier access to cannabinoid therapies and spurring further research and development in the field.

Integration of Cannabinoids in Traditional Medicine

Cannabinoids are increasingly being integrated into traditional medicine practices. This includes using cannabinoids as adjunct therapies in treatment regimens for chronic pain, cancer, epilepsy, and other conditions.

Focus on Safety and Quality Control

As cannabinoid use becomes more widespread, there is a growing focus on safety and quality control. This includes establishing standards for cannabinoid products, ensuring they are free from contaminants, and accurately labeled in terms of cannabinoid content.

Expanding Consumer Education

With the proliferation of cannabinoid products, there is an increasing need for consumer education. This involves informing the public about the benefits, risks, and appropriate use of cannabinoid products, helping consumers make informed decisions.

Cannabinoids in Veterinary Medicine

Emerging trends also include the use of cannabinoids in veterinary medicine. Pet owners and veterinarians are exploring the use of cannabinoids for treating various ailments in animals, from anxiety to pain management.

Sustainable Cultivation Practices

Sustainability in the cultivation of cannabis for cannabinoid production is becoming a more prominent concern. This includes adopting eco-friendly farming practices and exploring indoor cultivation methods that reduce environmental impact.

Global Market Expansion

The global market for cannabinoids is expanding rapidly. This growth is driven by increasing legalization, greater acceptance, and a wider recognition of the therapeutic potential of cannabinoids, leading to new opportunities in both medical and consumer markets.

Potential Challenges and Considerations

Despite these promising trends, challenges remain, including regulatory inconsistencies, the need for more extensive clinical trials, and addressing the stigma still associated with cannabis and certain cannabinoids like THC.

Conclusion

The emerging trends in cannabinoid use reflect a dynamic and rapidly evolving field. As scientific understanding grows and societal attitudes shift, cannabinoids are increasingly being recognized for their therapeutic potential and integrated into various aspects of healthcare and wellness. Navigating these trends responsibly will require ongoing research, education, and a commitment to safety and efficacy, paving the way for cannabinoids to make a significant impact on medicine and society.

www.ingramcontent.com/pod-product-compliance
Lightning Source LLC
Chambersburg PA
CBHW061008260726
48661CB00005B/2116